Caroline Sweeney is a reclusive and kind female whose experiences in life have left her broken, single, and unwanted in society. She now struggles with a medley of mental and other health problems that have culminated in schizophrenia. This is an inside-the-mind, brutally honest account of living with stigma, thinking with confusion, and the burden not just to herself but also to the siblings and parents who are part of her daily routine. It shows her complex relationship with invisible people, who are the only friends she has.

Thanks to my family for looking after me and helping me to do almost every chapter in this book. To the voices in my head... Thanks for listening in my darkest moments.

Caroline Sweeney

LIVING WITH THE VOICES OF WATCHERS AND HOPE

A Mental Illness Taboo

AUSTIN MACAULEY PUBLISHERS®

LONDON • CAMBRIDGE • NEW YORK • SHARJAH

A CIP catalogue record for this title is available from the British Library.

ISBN 9781035871797 (Paperback)
ISBN 9781035871803 (ePub e-book)

www.austinmacauley.com

First Published 2024
Austin Macauley Publishers Ltd®
1 Canada Square
Canary Wharf
London
E14 5AA

Early Intervention Team in Merseyside, you saved me. Merseyside Police, you were patient with me. Merseyside MPs and NHS staff, you supported me, thanks.

Table of Contents

I feel I have to put others at ease. I am tired of listening to 'opinions', albeit informed opinions, on a mental illness that none have personal experience of. Despite the information age expanding, some minds are still narrow in views. Stigma, media representation, and lack of available help (staff shortages, investment in treatments and pharmaceuticals), have led to an unseen epidemic of mental illnesses in society. Or at least a shameful taboo. Feeling humiliation and shame, schizophrenics, like myself, not only find it difficult to communicate with others but also be truthful with others about the things we hear. Doctors don't have the full picture.

What I
Wish to Achieve

I don't have much money to publish my story. So I am asking for your generosity.

I do not want payment for my story. I want any proceeds to be given by your publishing firm to mental health charities. My only personal request is that the 'Early Intervention Team' located at the South Sefton Neighbourhood Services, Waterloo, Merseyside would benefit from your gift. Please feel free to contact them and ask for Claire Verdin (a very wonderful care coordinator).

Personally, I want to help but I am afraid of bullies. I cannot contribute to the marketing of this book. That is making personal appearances. I will happily accept a representative from a charity. I can interact through them.

My parents, siblings, and my carers wholeheartedly support this publication. My voices are a little divided. My neighbours are none the wiser. The world – oblivious.

Thank you for your time, patience, and understanding. Best wishes to you and yours.

Yours Gratefully,

A Brief History of a Mental Society Old School Methods

The discovery of schizophrenia, according to mentalhelp.net, is reportedly attributed to a German psychiatrist Emil Kraepelin. He described the condition while treating people with symptoms in the late 1800s.

> DELUSIONS
> HALLUCINATIONS
> DISORGANISED THOUGHTS

He believed it was caused by an underlying 'brain disease'.

'BRAIN DISEASE?'

Yes, a 'brain disease' tha—

What? Something you catch?

Yes…

An 'infected mind'?

A 'brain disease'!

All right. Qualification does not make you an expert…

Yes, it does!

No, experience does! You know living on the inside of the condition, not a 'voyeur'!

The treatments before the 20th century, we can only guess.

No! We were oracles, witches, truth sayers, royalty. Everything from leeches and purging. What throwing up?

Exorcism, burning and prisons have been used to silence the voices, the demons, the…

YOU WHAT?

Twentieth-century treatments for schizophrenia include:

Insulin Coma Metrazol Shock (intravenous injections coma)

Electro Convulsive (electric shock)

Frontal Lobotomy (severing connections in the brain).

WHAT THE FUCK?

Hence, they are banned today.

I'm not fucking surprised.

In the 1950s, medication started to be used.

Thank fuck!

Now, 'talking therapies/CBT' are a trending 'low impact', be your own psychiatrist, methods with varying results for all mental illnesses.

Great…

What is difficult to determine is the exact number of schizophrenic deaths.

D-deaths? I hate you…

Due to these factors, according to the commons library.uk.

Geographic and economic factors, social/nationwide factors (e.g. COVID).

People who are never/not yet diagnosed (i.e. they are in denial and therefore do not seek help).

Mental illnesses are not recorded as a 'cause of death', or rather a 'direct cause of death' (other illnesses are also present like heart disease and diabetes).

What are you doing? You are scaring the poor readers. No, don't look! Let me handle this. Chances are the people reading this are my people.

Yes, my friends, we are here! Calling all loony-tunes young and wiser, you've heard from the dedicated doctors, now it's the aptly named patient's turn. Sorry about the voices. They do go on a bit not considering other people's feelings. So please read on and remember:

Don't take statistics as the gospel, because numbers lie.

All schizophrenics are still people, not serial killers.

And if things get desperate, you have rights. If you feel you are in danger or worried no one will believe you, you can contact healthcare professionals, even anonymously for help and reassurance.

I, Caroline, have thoughts of suicide. As a teen, I'd keep a backpack with clothing and essentials. Planned on either 'starting again' somewhere else or walking to the canal just across the field and throwing myself in with the rubbish. So please, please speak to someone online, on the phone, a local nurse, GP, or A&E consultant. I know you could wait a while but you are all worth it. Mental illness is not a sign of weakness. It's a sign to stop, talk, and listen. Please enjoy the book...

Our Caz and Schizophrenia
a Family

The Parents Story

Caroline, from a young age, had problems we didn't associate with her illness. She would hide under the kitchen tablecloth and quietly pull the chairs under. If you told her not to touch something, she would do it and then stay quiet or say it wasn't her.

My mum, Caroline's granny, took pride in the flowers in her back garden and waited ages for a particular flower to bloom. When it did, Caroline took all the petals off. When asked, Caroline said it wasn't her, it was the fairies. Maybe this was any child being mischievous, but none of our other children came close to not admitting anything.

She seemed to have a clue in her mannerisms. Caroline was quiet, had a good imagination, and had friends. There were no problems during infancy and early junior school. When she started secondary school, she became agitated. She'd get up early, walk in circles, and would not eat. We put it down to school pressures or maybe bullying. She wouldn't say. Then she began turning her back on visitors and facing the wall. She annoyed us but wouldn't tell us why she did it. She started to do this more frequently.

Then she started to write things in mid-air, nodding her head as if she was agreeing with someone or listening to someone. We asked her why she was doing it, but she wouldn't answer. Then we started finding pieces of paper around the house with symbols and religious quotes in her bed.

We also found she would hide other people's things like shoes or slippers. This happened when she was little, too. She tried flushing her brother's slippers down the toilet just because he argued with her.

Caroline left home to go to university where she had a breakdown. A breakdown we didn't get any explanation for until months later. We tried to find out from her, she wouldn't say, so we helped her as best we could. Her crying was part of the problem. It put us under stress because we didn't know what was the best way to help her.

She got a job and seemed happier. We thought it was because her mind was kept busy. After she started to become restless, getting up earlier than she should, and walking in circles. Then we had bad neighbours. They banged on walls at all hours. There was shouting, screaming, slamming doors, and playing loud music day and night.

Caroline tried to help everyone in the house by keeping it together and persevering. We tried to keep Caroline happy and tried not to let them stress her out. We got rid of the bad neighbours after they pestered her at work and we'd seen our local MP who was a great help.

Later, Caroline could still hear them banging on the walls, shouting her name and our names. She involved the police and got very argumentative with them. By now, we knew something had got worse with Caroline. My husband was in denial and refused to admit that Caroline needed help. When she was assessed, we had a feeling that maybe we should have done more to help her earlier on.

Caroline's whole identity changed from being happy and sure of herself. She questions every action she does and thinks. She's quiet most days, I don't know if it's her meds. Sometimes, there are glimpses of her but they quickly go.

She cries a lot and it stresses us out because we have to ignore her so she can work things out for herself. Most times she does. She talks about things she has experienced, what the voices say to her, or have said. We listen and try to swing the negative and upsetting things around so she understands what's wrong with what the voices say to her and try to make her see sense.

Caroline has tried to harm herself. She's talked about killing herself when the voices have really got to her. We all pull together to tell her that the voices aren't real and how much we love her. And not to listen to them. We are with Caroline nearly every minute of the day and night so she knows we are there for her.

It's hard, it's stressful to us and sometimes we feel like walking away for a few hours but we can't. Caroline is our daughter and her need is greater than ours.

The Early Intervention Team helped not just Caroline but us all as a family to cope. Sometimes we have falling outs but it's natural. It's our coping mechanism. They helped us understand more of what we were witnessing in Caroline's behaviour and understanding her mental illness.

Caroline can sometimes get angry but so do normal people and she copes really well. She will question her anger and other people's. We all have to listen closely to one another. It sometimes doesn't answer our questions, or maybe we don't like the answers, we are just humans and we can rub each other up the wrong way. It does blow over and it may take time but we all get there in the end.

Is it safe to put my head above the parapet? Hello?

Go away, Caroline. This isn't your section. People want to hear how your family feel about your illness. How they're coping.

(Rustling sound)
Caroline! What are you doing?
Trying to find my brothers' and sisters' bit.
Stop it! We don't want your influence here. Don't...
(Struggle taking place)
Give it back you crazy bitch! Stop trying to change words!
They don't understand! I need love!
(Smack)
Not-your-chapter! Get back to your own work!

Family Relations
Before and After

Family. A group of people with a close connection. We laughed together, lived together, and cried separately.

People tend to pass the blame like 'pass the parcel' (parlour game). I have varying degrees of loyalty and patience with family but I can honestly say that I both love and hate them equally. We easily put too much trust in them, which hurts more deeply if they let us down. Taking the blame, misdirecting the blame, or passing your mistakes off as other people's is more common than you think.

People are defined not by what they do but by the choices they make. Some are cowardly and selfish. Some are brave and selfless. All are judged by others. Family and what they think matters, doesn't it?

I never felt close to my mum for various reasons. She had me as a teenager. Teens are hormonal and unstable in thought and emotion. They are trying to find themselves. Children can change all that. Things happened. I just put it down to the 'my mum hates me' type of thing. Maybe she was depressed. Maybe I was jealous because she favoured my older brother (she came from a family of girls). Whatever the questions, Mum and I don't know the answers.

Naturally, Mum and Dad had a romantic courtship. It's warming to know. Mum for many years kept letters from Dad. They had run away together. Interesting romance but it's not my story to tell.

Dad had issues in his own life from Belfast to Liverpool. I love hearing his experiences, his stories, sad and funny. My dad is a strong character. He always deals with things 'head-on'.

When Dad was unemployed in the 80s we struggled. A lot of families on the council estates struggled. Families broke all over the place. Single parents everywhere. Debt, bailiffs, loan companies with extortionist interests, unpaid utilities, debt collector companies always knocking, getting essentials on tick if you were lucky and rented furniture became everyday life for a lot of us.

The 'family dynamic' kept changing over the years. I'd brought grief to my parents by them getting visited by the school board wanting to know why I had been skipping school. Bullying. I ended up looking after everyone and working, too. Couldn't afford my own home. Family comes first. People come and go but your parents and siblings, if you're lucky, will always shelter you from the worst the world has to offer.

When I broke, Dad took on the protector role but became too scared to ask me questions. Mum became more compassionate towards me and less angry. My siblings? Very strange. My brothers were behaving like nothing had changed. To them, I just got quieter. They had no 'beef' with me and would say so to my care coordinators from the Early Intervention Team during family sessions. My sisters? Completely different story.

"That's not my sister!" They didn't know who I was. We used to be so close doing funny dances, songs, nursery rhymes, crafts, games, or just talking. Now they don't know who I am? I felt betrayed, angry, and hurt. I prided myself on always being there for them. Now, when I needed understanding, I felt they weren't there for me. Feeling even more like an outsider, the word 'family' became sullied. It felt like there was a heavy and uncomfortable atmosphere that others noticed. Like walking slowly with a lit stick of dynamite. Everyone and the voices were pointing at me. I always thought 'bad people' win. No one gets closure. Just get on with it…my sisters don't love me anymore.

They either don't remember the things we did or just cut me off. People fear what they don't understand. I wanted to make happy memories. Keep them innocent for as long as possible because the world was cruel enough. What use is a memory with no one to share them with?

How do I fix this?

Ploughing my mind with numbing family therapy and reading about my schizophrenia, if I could concentrate, I am still confused but somewhere along all the chaos, I shut down. I began to see the voices as family. They know me. They listen. When you're in a deep, dark place, an emotional abyss, the tears stop. When medical people ask me if I think the voices are real, I say no. I am lying. I'm afraid of being put in the 'loony bin'. Just saying someone isn't there doesn't change the fact that I can hear them or see them. The voices, despite trying to kill me early on, have proved to be the longest 'relationship' I have ever had.

They are funny and scary at the same time. They call me a "retarded woman" but offer to listen to me when no one else will. Funny faces, policing my mind. You cannot tell me that love and hate are separate. Extreme emotion usually makes me 'push away' people under the family umbrella. The voices won't leave me no matter how angry I get, how ugly I am, or how confusing I can be. Is that what family is?

But don't get any wrong ideas about my siblings or parents. We will keep trying to fix ourselves and each other. I am not dead yet.

Recollections that occurred to me as I did this section:

I'm about five years old. Clarabel (a large pink teddy) and Scrappy (a small lime green puppy toy) are in my arms. I am downstairs after having nightmares. Dad was asleep on the sofa. I thought if I went back to sleep by myself then there would be more nightmares. So, rubbing my eyes with my toys hugged against me, I woke Dad and then slept on the sofa with him.

Looking out of the living room window, as a small child, I saw a pony in the next door's driveway. It was my friend's birthday. I couldn't join them because I'd just recovered from chickenpox. As I was just getting over my bout, my older brother came down with it. I just watched.

To King, Smokey, Joey, Tramp, Ross, Spicy and Brandy. From a dog that thought he was a cat climbing curtains. A crazy pup that would pee on my brother when I told him to (soz). To two beautiful tortoiseshell cats. One very dark and quiet. The other was a bright white patchwork crazy. I miss you all. Even though you only knew me for a short time (why were they deprived of knowing me?). Do pets know if you have mental problems?

Childhood games, no computer, only four channels, no money. Hide and seek, rhyming games (like Dan, Dan the-man), eating grass, hopscotch, shark attack, sleeping lions and creating our own board games...or was that just me?

Be crazed because laughter keeps you sane, well saner...I think.

Definition of a 'family':

A measurable unit or group of species that live in close proximity to each other.

Or

A 'normal' social nexus of habitual living that works together to progress their species.

Or maybe this

The reason you're happy/miserable (according to Freud).

I do not believe my 'family' or 'family umbrella' are responsible for my schizophrenia. It's a combination of stupid stuff. Like chapters in a book, a ripple in the water or an echo in a cave. Hereditary? Maybe, but I am the problem. Maybe I am the cause. Maybe it's through the choices I made good and bad. If stress was a factor, how we deal with the fallout tests our resiliency as individuals, it would define us.

Family is not the cause, it should be a 'coping mechanism'. And as a cog in a well-oiled, colourful, weirdo machine, all my family and family umbrellas know that we will be the untrained listeners. The bottomless wallet, well, a coin purse. The roof over our heads, and a major league 'pain in each other's butts'.

Keep family diaries of thoughts and feelings, both positive and negative. In a year's time, look at them, and share them. You've come a long way, baby!

Mental illness shouldn't mean you can't create happy memories. Schizophrenics and depressives don't want to be remembered as a 'burden'. Who knows? Putting the effort in on both sides could not only help to cope but create a silver lining. Reading the latest best sellers or poetry, ahem, whatever the genre, to each other, could bring people back together. Personally, I love Keats, Byron, Dawn French and classic B-movies and Whodunits. Hell, turn the TV on and pick a horse in the next race. I'll have two packets of Maltesers and a packet of biscuits on the first favourite. See which horse goes past the finishing post first.

I'm putting all my jam marshmallows on 'Jam's Bond'!

The jammies? Are you crazy? Oh, sorry you are. Well, it's your sugar coma!

Reminiscing with life experiences, even cringe-worthy ones, is our brain's natural tonic. If you want to be cruel, break out the photo albums. If you want to be a pain in the arse to unwilling participants, break out the projector, slides, and laser pointers and stream it all live on the Tube.

Talk about current affairs. Put the world to rights. Don't wait for the silence to take hold. Being trapped in your own mind is giving up. The only person you are talking to is yourself. And if you are assaulted with negative thoughts and emotions, is that the person you should be listening to?

'The Patience of Angels' isn't just a song, it's an achievement. Please take your time. I know that there's a lot

to be done, you all have your own lives to live, and your own families to tend to. You are, you were, and you will always be loved and appreciated for that. Any time well spent isn't time wasted. Thanks, family!

A little theatrical, isn't it?

Oh, piss off! If you don't like it, don't read it…Bitch.

Why are you so aggressive?

Why are you looking for a fault? I am angry at this moment because you are ignoring the positive things I've just expressed and are pushing the negative.

Isn't that what you do?

You mean that I remember the negative more than the positive memories?

Yes!

No…Well, maybe a bit. Am I who I think I am? Or what others think I am?

You're in your 40s now and you still don't know who you are?

I hear different things.

Are you a 'bad person' or a 'good person'?

I wouldn't want anyone to feel bad unless they are 'bad'. I try to make 'good' choices based on the situation. I wouldn't leave my worst enemy crying in the street. But I do not want to be a carpet for 'abusive' people either. If I keep my head down, if I remain quiet, not bother anyone then maybe the 'bad people' won't see me. I'm a ghost.

The Voices Story

This may not be a good idea but they are going to share their story. Go on, tell the nice readers why you liked to eff with my mind.

I do not understand how you feel ten times the emotion that we do. Your younger self behaves similarly. (Discussion; lots of voices talking)

We do live opposite you. We still miss you. (A different voice interrupts) *Caroline, don't think of us. Think of your own experience.*

(Busy voices. Arguing?)

We can't talk about ourselves. We can ask you questions but that's it.

Is that a rule you have to follow?

That is a rule we choose to follow. We can't make sense of you. Your mind is a different life altogether. You can't fit into your world, you remove yourself from it. Explain it to us.

At this point, I stopped typing what they said. They were probing me and my past in a vulgar way. I felt they were attacking me. It's none of their business. I have the right to some 'privacy'.

NOTE: My siblings don't feel comfortable making their experiences of my schizophrenia public. I will respect that decision and their privacy.

Explaining Me: Understanding the Person Behind the Schizophrenia

Okay, so I don't know if it's schizophrenic but I'm always explaining. Mainly what I've said or written, maybe writing it is the same as saying it, I think. For example:

Caz: "The cat's out!" (Silence)

Caz: "The...cat's out!"

(Silent nodding and people looking at me)

Caz: "I just let the cat out. He wanted out. He was pawing at the door."

(Brief pause)

Caz: "I think he's after the birds...you know, the fat one. The one we inflamed 'Christmas dinner'. That one. You know..."

(One hour later)

Caz: "Cat! He's in. Must have been chasing birds. Probably the big one."

(Silence)

Caz: "I'm sure it's teasing him..."

Strangely, I seldom get told to 'shut up'. Probably because we are all shut up in different ways. An enclosed space. Rolled into a ball of anxieties. In fact, shutting up is natural. People shut up all the time. It's a matter of choice, really. I mean we can shut up or shut down. No matter how you see each task they both mean silence in the end. So yeah, I can shut up, shut down…as opposed to 'open up' or 'open down' but even then I…Voices just told me to 'shut up' again. *Shhhhh…rude.*

So when I confronted the voices I used different forms of communication. "Don't worry, I speak the language." Charades, well writing words in mid-air with my right index finger, while getting strange looks that I was completely unaware of.

Sometimes, I air drew pictures. Mock all you want, I could've won awards for that bit of modern art. But, being philistines, the most successful form of communication is …thinking.

Therefore, I came to the conclusion that either I was a psychic or my neighbours had taken up ventriloquism. A possibility. But no one could hear these voices but me. Scary.

The voices told me that they were communicating with me, and others, via brain waves. Turning waves into words via an earpiece. Later, I saw an article in Geographic about an AI hearing aid that allowed the deaf to hear working at a similar principle. Cool, I knew I was afraid of tech for a reason.

Doctors think that schizophrenics use the listening/speech part of the brain when the voices are present. Yet we still can't account for all of our brain's functions. Except me. My brain function is to seek out and find pizza no matter what the cost.

Whatever the topping, I'm there. Whatever the side order, I'm there. Whatever the amount, they can all fuck off it's mine!

I don't think that some of the male voices agree with me over anything. Maybe they think I'm weird. Females are the cattiest, most of them. They can all be cruel, uncaring, shallow bullies. Bullies I can't walk away from. They are always there. Here or there? Feel the same. I cry a lot. I cried a lot. I have one wall mirror in my home, in the living room. What I see in there varies through the day; I've been known to scream.

I like people's wrinkles. Like a root, branches, a diary. They show what kind of life you have had. Positive emotions, negative ones. Lines can change, and increase but your eyes are always the same. I used to think that I could one day gaze into my partner/friend's eyes and, with my fingertips, trace every line they have. Smile at the happy ones and kiss away the sad ones. That won't happen for me. My face is a road map to hell. I'm not evil. I'm in a constant state of confusion. I don't notice people at the moment. I can't be noticed.

I've spent my entire life with one question: Why? The reasons are too much for me to explain. Someone made me feel wrong. While other people, bad and good, have grown, had long-term relationships, have families of their own, and bettered themselves, I'm the last one. I have myself…oh, and the voices. I think my parents and siblings question whether I'm the problem.

Bullies move on, do the victims?

I still feel like facing the corner of the room, begging people not to look at me. I must be offensive in some way. A lot of bad experiences in my life and I am the only common denominator. So here I am alone, unloved, barren, overweight, depressed, losing my hair, and coping with schizophrenia.

Laugh-it-up!

Stop explaining why you're a 'retarded woman'. Shut up!

I never grew up thinking about kids, marriage, relationships, being a boss or a friend. I just wanted to make it through the day.

The voices represent my worst fears...two extremes. Sephiroth and Arbiters. Half angel, half demon. An entity that, at my request, negotiated a plea for me between heaven and hell. I was desperate. I didn't want my family harmed in any way. I'd already broken down. All my fight had gone. I was afraid that I couldn't protect them. But everything has a price, whatever happened to them the negativity aimed at me would be at least three-fold. You can't ask for bad things to happen and have no consequences. So the voices behaved accordingly.

It threatened my siblings, trapped me with child abusers only I could see and hear, raped me, encouraged me to seriously hurt people around me and harm myself. I couldn't tell people what they said. Why? Sicko, loony bin. Justification for other people's hatred and ignorance. I'm not a bully or abuser. Why would my own mind do that to me? That is not me! I had to protect my siblings, parents, nephews and co-workers from this 'nightmare' as the voices would say in their own words 'bastardising' me.

It took a leap of faith to trust anyone. What I heard or saw made me physically sick. Could I talk about it to anyone?

I was in turmoil opening up to the Early Intervention Team. I believed people would say I'm having bad hallucinations because I'm a bad person. I don't want to hurt anyone. I don't ever want to be coerced, or forced to hurt anyone. The voices made me feel like a 'monster'. I felt weak. The team told me I wasn't weak and agreed that the voices were merely my worst fears come true. At least mentally.

At this point in time, talking with my voices, I still can't remember how to do my job in a ladies' clothes shop, but I am spiritually in a better place. I'm not grinding my teeth, always on edge. The voices' aggressive bullying tactics caused the stress I had already 'cracked up' with to become worse. My stress bucket overflowed with stuff. More hours, less contracted hours, no pension, bad neighbours, keeping the family sane and happier, trying to stay positive. Housing saying stuff isn't their problem, police saying there is nothing they can do, back to the housing, keeping anti-social diaries, keeping in contact with our MP and being overwhelmed by anti-social people in work, including my bad neighbours...now I began seeing people, hearing people that I couldn't get away from 24 hours a day. I wanted to die. But the bastards wouldn't give me that.

So I was forced to pull out of work until I was 'better'. Worked with my family and the Intervention Team to gain some sanity. I hadn't realised how fast my thoughts were until someone pulled the plug. My mind didn't feel right. I felt like a passenger seeing through someone else's eyes. Everything suddenly stopped...darkness, blackout, and confusion. I forgot everything and just heard people telling me I was the problem. So I agreed.

They told me they watched me in the shower. That I'm a 'monster' not a real woman. Some voices even told me they were child abusers and as well as abusing me, they threatened to abuse my younger siblings by talking to them. No one else heard them. But if I could, so could they. Couldn't they? I secretly rubbed bleach into my skin to try to feel clean. Pulled at my hair. Stole other people's pain medication. Cried and scratched what I could, hoping that people wouldn't notice.

Sorry…that was unexpected. Did the voices show remorse? Anyone who has ever harmed me has never apologised, let alone meant it. It sounded sincere.

I'd been talking mentally non-stop. I thought that if I told them everything I'd ever experienced no matter how mundane, they would know the truth and leave. Leave me alone. They stayed and confused me. More nicer one minute than nasty the next. It was a form of torture. They'd lull me into thinking they were genuinely sorry, then when I trusted them with a bit more personal information, they'd dig the image in deeper. All the while, I had become silent to everyone around me.

As I've mentioned before, I don't trust people. I'd rather walk away from people or run from them. I just can't understand why bad people, young and old, feel no remorse. I only have to argue or confront someone and later I feel…less.

There is a voice I called (funny face). He seemed to want to understand me. Made me laugh and offered some protection at the risk of his own mind. Not like me. I'm a coward but I know that. He brought me hope and comfort in the sterile room I'd been locked up in. I was naked. I had burnt wings. Chained up in an observation room he bandaged my bloodied hands. At the window, familiar faces stared in but never did anything else.

Everything stopped.

So I live like a recluse these days. I'm schizophrenic but you 'normal' people scare me. I'd rather face a wall than a mirror. Always looking for an exit. As a coward, I react to people, I don't instigate.

They say only a truly desperate man turns to God as the last resort. I have prayed more to God than I ever have. I slept with a Bible under my pillow. Hoping that it would keep the 'nightmare' away, I held it just as tightly as a little girl holding a lime green, cuddly puppy.

In these times, we are finding that good and evil aren't as straightforward as we'd like. Maybe that confusion allows the 'bad' to feel good and the 'good' to feel bad about themselves.

Still explaining yourself? They've stopped listening.

I still believe I'm a burden to everyone. Taking other people's time and energy. Honestly, I expected the voices to have left me by now. I must be boring by now or so annoying they'd run screaming. I push people away because I'm afraid of making them feel my misery (like the girl crying at a party). We all have a 'mad woman in the attic'. I just sit and talk to mine.

I am not stupid. I choose not to hurt anyone. I'm not dangerous. My mental illness stems from my very worst fears. Everything is happening to me. I'm just afraid because no one can help. Hope is a constant, it is always there.

Schizophrenics are emotional rollercoasters. Medicines and treatments give hope to sufferers. A step in the right direction. Take this one day, one step, and one action at a time. You're braver than you think.

Schizophrenics are not serial killers! We are siblings, parents, friends, and neighbours, even loners. It's choices that determine who we are, not whether we 'fit in'.

Finding Solutions

One day...

I directed a question to my psychiatrist...

"How do I prove it?"

Other 'norms' assume that people who hear voices are lying. Or weak-minded and on something. What the doc conjectured (you're not impressing anyone) was that research was ongoing.

But how does schizophrenia affect our bodies?

Angry voices = Blood pressure, increased heart rate

Kind voices = Increased brain activity, extra energy

Could technology help people with schizophrenia? Cure dementia? Inhibit cancers?

Medications for Schizophrenics
(I Don't Bloody Know)
Or They Said It Not Me
(You Still Typing?) No

Do not be afraid of the term 'aunty psychotic' because there is no such thing. 'Antipsychotics' are real, although I've never seen them.

Caroline…Caroline?

Okay. Medicine is serious, buoys and gills. *Happy?*

Yes. I am.

These medicines are, mostly, non-invasive…I can feel his eyes burning into the back of my head. We've come a long way, should've taken the school route. Would've got there quicker. I…er-ahem…no? Meds these days are good and can only get better. However, availability and rising costs could prevent people from getting the help they need.

Dear Pharma Company,

As people around the world try to cope with the modern world they, though strong in spirit, need your help to repair their body and mind. As the number of people with mental illnesses grows, your dedicated workers offer hope to millions. Every new discovery is a godsend. But:

The cost of drugs and treatments means that our 'coping' depends upon affordability.

In turn, the availability of medicines worldwide should mean not one price for all but 'prices based on global income'.

Governments need to invest in mental health drug research and work with agencies and charities to understand the cost of production and the cost of distribution.

Make more age-appropriate medicines, in earth-friendly ways and reduce the stigma surrounding illnesses and the taking of medication.

Explore any potential long-term effects of medicine alone or with alternative treatments.

Apart from that, you're grand! Thank you.

Signed,

Schizo Phrenic ABC, 123, BAD; ASS

My own prescription:

Propranolol = anti-anxiety

Quetiapine = antipsychotic

Sertraline = antidepressant

Others that I've had:

Aripiprazole = antipsychotic (less side effects)

Procyclidine = combats the side effects of other medication

I feel bad about how much my meds cost the NHS.

Taxpayers keep me alive. Thank you. There is no way I could ever afford these medicines.

These meds didn't 'cure' my schizophrenia but they helped me cope physically.

CBT is an ongoing thing that can help you realise you aren't 'evil' or feel 'ashamed' about what goes on in the confused battle inside you.

Together, these things offer you the best chance of living a more 'normal' life. Maybe you're the lucky one that is cured. Be a mental health 'survivor'.

Schizophrenia is relentless. There is no holy grail. Sorry. But, we do have hope that it will get easier.

Pharmacy companies are the future. People are living longer but population growth, longevity, age-related illnesses, and new epidemics need economic stability and an increased 'quality of life' to succeed long-term.

The industrial revolution earmarked British history. Surely, the era of medicinal reparation and the understanding of benign tech for the care of others is advantageous to everyone.

Obviously, someone would abuse this tech research for negative profit or war machines (short-term money-makers). But an inhibitor, a microchip booster to bolster memories, confuse cancers, or silence the voices would free trapped people. Give them hope.

We are a diverse planet with diverse species. The human brain is still such a mystery despite all of our tech advances and know-how. If we can aid those in need, what we discover could help other species on this planet. Mental health and its impact on society is a far-reaching problem and solutions can benefit everyone e.g. First settlers on Mars coping mentally.

Let's share solutions to social problems all over the world. If other countries were safe and prosperous, there wouldn't be a migrant crisis, overpopulation, and conflicting economic factors. If people were cared for, safe, made fair trade deals, and cancelled world debt, they wouldn't put other countries under strain. Take your money for war and, even for one year, give it to those in your country who need your help. Every business, celebrity, or politician who makes over a certain amount, how about once every five years give back to the community you came from? Anything from donating to local schools and charities to building homes for the homeless and providing food to those less fortunate.

Let's make all people safer. Make sure no one is left behind. Fair deals on medication, help where needed despite the cost, and information to make every life matter. I vote for the 'Florence Nightingale Effect'. Protect our future kin and become heroes, not just role models. Shine a light in the dark and keep watch at their bedside.

Please, a whisper is more important than a shout. Mental health is important to understand, identify, and choose. I cannot curse future generations of my family tree into a hereditary nightmare. So here I am as a whisper to help us.

#PharmaSafePlaceMindSpace2023

DON'T BE AFRAID TO ASK MENTAL HEALTH QUESTIONS.

Venture a simple question and see if people open up. If they choose not to, don't worry, they just don't feel comfortable answering yet. They will, however, appreciate you because you asked. Asking about any concerns you have is better than worrying. Just chat. Alternatively, approach family, carers, charities and ask them. Always be respectful. Don't flaunt your prejudices.

My Traveller Friend Amanda
I Wish You Well

In the 1980s, Amanda and her parents moved around frequently.

I saw her all alone and looking sad in the playground. Another friend at the time came up to me and asked me to play with our usual group of friends. Feeling bad for her, I'd asked my friend if Amanda could play with us, too. My arm was grabbed and two other girls joined us.

"She's not playing." They pointed at Amanda.

Honestly, I really considered joining my friends. Instead, I walked up to Amanda and asked if she wanted to play with me. Amanda looked nervously towards the others. So I saved her the choice and stayed with her. She seemed interesting.

Over the course of her time at Thornton, I learnt more about her. She'd been to lots of different schools and she said she didn't have friends. To begin with, she'd tell me to, "Go away!" But I'm an annoying pain in the arse so I stayed with her, followed, and talked to her. I think I wore her down. We would always have breaks and dinner together. I don't recall what the others thought. It's okay if Amanda didn't want to play with them. I don't think they liked her. Shame, they missed out.

However, one day, she wouldn't say a word to me. Every time I approached her, she walked away with her back to me. At lunch, I usually held a seat for her. The hall was packed and a dinner lady asked to put me at a table with my classmates.

Believing that Amanda, for some reason, hated me, I agreed.

Hurriedly tucking into dinner, I saw Amanda enter and look around. She looked like she'd cry. Another dinner lady asked her if she wanted to sit with her friend. She looked over at me and shook her head. The lady then sat her at another table. No one spoke to her. I tried to approach her in the playground afterwards but she walked away.

In my own self-involved head, I was wondering what I'd done. I rushed to the toilets, sat in a cubicle and cried. Trying to catch my breath, I heard a thudding sound at my door. Feeling dizzy, I sat on the floor and went quiet. Eventually, I think it was the dinner lady who found me, asked me to wash my face and go back to lessons.

By afternoon break, I was angry. I stood in front of Amanda and asked her why she didn't like me anymore. Still just thinking about myself. She looked shocked and then whispered. Basically, she was leaving. Another school, another country, and she didn't want to tell me. She was gone the next day. Another brave person. I don't know where she is but I hope she found her smile...for someone who said she had no friends she certainly has at least one.

After this, I began distancing myself from the others in my year. Didn't trust them in the end but I didn't realise this until high school.

On that note, I do not have a passport. I am not a wandering schizo. I wish I could see places like Florence, Mauritius, or Copenhagen. I have read books, seen documentaries, and gazed at artwork inspired by these places all from an armchair. Why? Because I don't feel safe in public places, mainly crowded ones. People make me feel awkward. I run away. I barely look up. Afraid to attract negative attention. I work on the assumption that people don't like me. They don't like my name, my skin colour, my alopecia – I'm just wrong. I don't fit in. I feel constantly judged and ridiculed because I am.

I cannot sit for a passport interview because I struggle with going over things and answering what should be simple questions. I misinterpret questions or I can't hear the interviewer. Their lips are moving but I can't take it in. People get frustrated with me. The passport office is in town. Lots of traffic, people, worries, and voices. Just waiting for the lift home is stressful.

The more nervous I am, the more accident-prone I get. On my first day at work, I flooded the kitchen destroying signs, tickets etc. My first week, I threw out the rubbish and, how did that happen, I ended up in the bin myself. Security thought I jumped. They could have helped me out. Those bins are deep. And when it came to whether my boss was going to keep me on after a trial, I nearly concussed her. The till drawers were spring loaded and my manager (who is a lovely person) bent down to get a till roll from under my till, which happened to still be there when I completed a sale. DING! BONK! The drawer shot out so fast and with such force, that my manager (a very kind person), fell backwards in a heap.

Probably didn't help that we had a queue and we were only two on tills…She kept me on.

So being accident-prone on aeroplanes or in foreign countries where the locals and staff may not be trained for people like me, could lead to a diplomatic incident. Or the voices and I will more than likely get lost and end up in the North Pole with the locals. So I'm afraid I'll have to pass on the passport…tumbleweed.

A Tina

Tina had a profound effect on me. A naturally ombre brown/blonde who is beautiful inside and out. A bright spark. This girl made exams look effortless. Very kind and courteous (she had a badge to prove it).

Tina was picked on by boys from the juniors onward. Some would call her names like 'half-cast' but both parents were white. I didn't realise what was happening to her but I had been a witness to some of it.

She had a focused mind. I was in awe of her in high school. She was in the chess club, choir, cadets, and art club and loved Morris dancing with Caledonians (like cheerleading). She also played a couple of instruments including a flute. Always busy. I didn't understand why people wouldn't like her. She was interesting and funny.

In contrast, I was annoying, a decent singer, enjoyed drawing, pretty daring at draughts, published at an early age, annoying, funny, dirty humour, fart obsessed and annoying. Did I mention annoying?

Talking about yourself again, Caroline. Focus.

Tina's exams were faultless. I remembered, witnessed, and spoke to her about how she handled bullying. She told me, "One day at a time." Her words stuck with me all these years.

During our GCSEs, in breaks, we went to McD's in Crosby. I had no money but wanted the company. Tina ordered and we sat at a table so she could eat. The place was full. Lots of families, lots of noise. The table across from us was full of lads.

They began targeting us.

"Milk bottle", weird animal impersonations, the 'N' word. I struggle to recall the other things. I forget what I heard but remember the emotions, still feel them.

They threw fries at Tina and I, bits of bun. They were yelling at us. I was frightened and looked around at families and staff but no one helped us even though they were all looking. I was crying when we left but Tina seemed so calm. She even stopped to speak to her aunt she'd spotted outside.

Such a positive person despite being surrounded by negativity. Something in common? I can hope.

Tina wanted to become a police officer. I hope she did. We need people like her. An unwavering moral compass that isn't influenced by the authority of others. When negative things get too much for me, I ask for courage and strength. I think it looks like Tina. Thank you, T!

They closed that particular McD's soon after because the staff couldn't cope with the troublemakers. Also, they had a notice that said school kids could only come in if accompanied by an adult.

No one else will see you either. I don't know the answer.

Self-Loathing Sadness

Depression is a dark, deep, and silent abyss.

Schizophrenia and depression are scary stuff. It's like being locked in a windowless room and being forced to listen to negativity on a loop in various unrecognisable voices. All alone. Silenced by bombardment. You stop speaking. Soon you stop feeling. Surprisingly, you begin to tune in to your own whispering voice. Mea culpa. All my fault.

Snap out of it.

I can't!

You can!

If I could, I would have done it by now.

Other people don't let it bother them.

Am I weak?

Maybe.

I did not 'choose' to be depressed. I have no control.

What reason do you use to excuse your sadness?

My rent is paid for me. I am on benefits that take care of my bills. Benefits offer me some kind of inclusion in a society that sees me as a psycho and a sponger. An underclass loon that should be locked up for being different and forgotten.

Nobody deserves abuse. But kids, as well as adults, are perpetrators and victims. Did I ask to be bullied? Because I saw no one else suffering. Is it me? Really? My fault? My fault. What is it about me you hate so much? Why are you and your friends, 'cause I don't have any, laughing and happy at seeing me suffer?

Nobody else was pushed against the railings, harassed, gossiped about, and ridiculed in the street as well as in the classroom. Why are they laughing? Am I too different?

I'm sorry, does my distress bother you?

It's the past. Move on. You're being oversensitive.

So I'm the one with the problem?

They've just grown up with problems. If we all show understanding, trust and care about them, maybe they'll treat people better. So they are the victims? I am so sorry. I foolishly thought the terrible things they did was their inability to distinguish right from wrong. I'm sorry. Please, sir, may I have another? When they called me a "sad bitch" in front of the class, I should have fucking hugged them. If I wasn't such a freak, forcing their young minds to treat me badly and abuse me, they'd be better people.

How dare I breathe the same air.

You forgot the question mark.

It was RHETORICAL!

Deep breath…

I feel like an old piece of china. A dusty teacup. I have been dropped, thrown and knocked over so many times that people get sick of trying to glue me back together. After a while, people only see the cracks. They give up. Throw it out. It was on the shelf too long anyway.

As a teen, I was so badly bullied I'd stand facing the corner of the living room. Often crying. Sometimes repeating in a shaky voice I didn't recognise as my own, "Do not look at me, I'm ugly", "My face offends people", "There's something wrong with me". No one told me that I was wrong, I probably wouldn't believe them anyway.

I'd zone out. Staring at nothing or looking at life outside the window. If you concentrate hard enough, then you can't see anything else.

All those bullies must have felt justified because they never said "sorry". It was always my fault. They didn't seem to target many other people, if any. I've no closure. In my mind, it's not over. They were never punished. I was never helped. Years later, the abuse is still going on in my head.

ANGER?

I got so angry as a teen I threatened to kill my family in their sleep. I was screaming so loudly that nobody heard me. What I said hurt like a knife or a razor, dragged across my heart and stabbed as a reminder. I am still sickened with myself to this day. I chose to say it. I'm sorry. I really am so sorry.

Your choices.

Yes. I wanted to kill myself. I tried – perhaps not hard enough. Trying to overdose on my parent's prescription painkillers. Stood on the edge of a canal. Rubbed bleach into my skin. Rubbing my eyes. I'm a coward. Failure. The most sickening part is I am still here. Other people, good people, who deserved to live have been robbed of life by cancer, by crime, by hate, by fear. Why not me? Do you deserve to die?

'Druggie', 'lesbian' or maybe 'weirdo' – I love that. I am not a 'norm'. 'LIAR' – that word again. Why do people want to believe everything negative? Why am I only lying if I am recalling positive things? Do you feel your abuse is justified if you want to believe the negative? God forbid that you are a bully!

Sometimes I was happy that I was good at something.

Would you be less scathing if someone else was as good as them? Real friends would be happy for me, and supportive. Instead, I even apologised for it. I let them abuse me without a fight and they still couldn't accept me…It is me, isn't it? I am not complete.

Get over it, Caroline. Move on.

I will slap the next person who says that to anyone with a mental illness.

So those trying to help are a problem too? Isn't that being oversensitive to constructive criticism?

Why? Because I finally found the guts to stand up for myself?

People see you differently. The world doesn't revolve around you. Your thoughts, your memories, your feelings. Are yours the only ones that matter?

There is so much chaos and confusion inside me. The conflict has to stop. All I want is silence.

What happened as an adult?

In my mid-twenties, my life stopped. We had 'bad neighbours'. I heard and saw some fucked up shit. Sexualisation of school kids, a mother who was a neglectful alcoholic drug dealer, shoplifting, a mum that supplied alcohol to, not only her own children but also other people. A prolific liar who manipulated everyone into believing that she

49

was the real victim of it all. "She's had a bad life." She chose. She knew doing all those things was wrong so why choose to do them? There are many families in the same situation but they chose the right things to protect their children, protect others. She got all the help but no punishment. That'll stop her from doing it again. That'll teach those kids to do better for themselves (outraged sarcasm). Went to court, all on public record.

Finished? The past? Feel and move on.

This was the final nail in my coffin. I was emotionally, physically, spiritually, and mentally burnt out. I was working through all this. Kept in close contact with our local MP. Tried to give my siblings time and attention because I was worried about how they felt. I cracked.

I, embarrassingly, cracked at work. Recently, I'd begun hearing other people. It was at night at first. Then while at work then at home. Getting louder and louder to the point where I heard them like they were sitting next to me. The things they said were horrific and eventually, I stopped interacting with everyone. I was separating myself. I felt dirty and tainted. I felt violated. It felt like a memory. I didn't want to contaminate the kids. Said nothing. Just prayed. At some point, the bleach couldn't clean me enough. I couldn't get up.

The voices threatened to do the same to my younger siblings. In what I thought was my last breath, I phoned the police at work threatening to kill myself. Minutes later, the police arrived at my workplace. Probably thought I was a loony. Are you laughing at me? Would you laugh if your family member said this?

Bullies and abusers, even if caught, they get looked after. They have a rush of people offering to do things for them.

Once a victim brings those people to the attention of people I trust, everyone leaves, turns the light off, and goes home, thank you. You're just left with the voices. Collective whispering…

Looking Back at
the Signs

Hearing Things Others Didn't

The 'bee incident'. My bed was right next to a ventilation hole for the boiler in our family's home. Day and night, I would hear buzzing. Nobody else did. I kept twitching or running from the room scared but no one else ever heard the buzzing.

I was very scared. If I was terrified, then I wouldn't be able to move. Something would happen if I moved, but if I saw an escape route, I was going for it.

Anyway, I would get upset that no one else heard it. Then one day a large, almost hornet-like bee came out of the vent and into the room. I called Mum to show her. She let it out as its buzzing became aggressive. She then banged the wall with her hand and listened closely to the wall. Every time we tapped the wall there, we heard buzzing. *Finally, they can hear it! I'm not crazy.*

A man came out to investigate it. Yes, bees confirmed. He said they weren't aggressive no matter how close he got. Fair enough.

The voices? Oh, many years ago as a teen, in my bed under the light, I woke in the early hours to hear a voice say, "Sit up".

Half asleep, I responded, "No".

Then an imperious male voice demanded, "Get up NOW!" I do not know why but I sat bolt upright. I heard a clunk and felt something brush the top of my head and a thud on the bed behind me. It was the light bulb.

It happened again, the same male voice when I was a teen back from university. I woke up frozen. Extremely cold and frightened. It felt like a heavy arm was lying across my chest and what I think was a leg lying across mine. I couldn't move. I heard heavy breathing, a man's like he was asleep next to me. I couldn't speak. In my head, I asked him to leave because I was frightened. I didn't know what was happening. So in my head, I begged him to leave and to prove he was real, so he would say my name. A deep, sleepy, breathy voice said my name into my left ear. I repeated that I was scared. Again, I asked him to leave. He did. I started to feel warmth in my toes. Then feet. Only when it reached my chest, could I draw a deep breath and move.

Part of me wishes I'd asked his name now. In hindsight, he wasn't scary. It felt protective. I should have been braver.

I do remember strange clocks. I love clocks, except digital ones, their high-pitched alarms make me jump and fill me with dread. I'd wake, intermittently, worrying about getting up for school. I would sneak into my parents' room and turn off the alarm. Years later, I found out that my brother would sometimes do the same. Silent, like ninjas or Jedi. No, we stick with the ninja.

There was a digital clock on something in my room at bed height. One night, I woke up and looked at the clock. Instead of numbers, the actual word, 'SLEEP' was displayed. You'd think that would wake me right up. No! I went back to sleep.

Again, towards the end of our 'bad neighbours', along with multiple voices, I began to see strange things:

A beam of green light seemed to come from the bedroom wall between the neighbours and us.

Shadows in the garden.

Moving lights in carrier bags on the field that would disappear at the thicket of thorns.

Men dressed either all in white or all in black. Later it was just men/a blonde man in just black that no one else sees.

Spiders crawling.

Bad Neighbours
the Swines

When I Cracked Up (Became a Schizo-Bitch)

Okay! This, like me (according to the voices), won't be pretty. Forewarned! These people made me what I am today: Almost silent, unhappy, appalled, and sarcastic (maybe not the last one).

One day a neighbour, who didn't see eye to eye with their other neighbour (who didn't like anyone and blamed others), moved to 'Tin Town'. They swapped with the worst 'family' they could find to upset their nosy neighbour. It was bad from the get-go.

First day! The mother disappeared ASAP. The 'kids', who never would have gone to school if we hadn't insisted, were alone. Loud music, and swearing that would make a prostitute blush, coupled with weed, cigarettes and copious amounts of alcohol, that were given to them by their mother before she buggered off. Stop me if I get too technical. This bullshit is horrible to think about let alone bare my soul.

Drunken arguing is how this 'family' communicated with each other. That night, the police were called because her teenage lad, who we later found out was possibly older, and his little sister, who we thought was fourteen but turned out to be twelve, coerced kids they didn't even know to enter their new home and plied them with alcohol and drugs. When the police insisted on calling the mother, her 'responsible' young son reluctantly rang her and the problem Mum asked the other neighbour, "Do I have to?" The kids that were there, whom her son and daughter couldn't name, had lied to their parents about where they were, their parents had no idea about the alcohol; and the police officer, while sympathetic, told us, "At least they are doing it in their own homes, not out on the street."

He completely missed the point! They were underage. They shouldn't be drinking in the first place. Why weren't those kids' parents asked if they wanted to take action against this 'family'? Why were their children given drugs and alcohol to the point where one of them vomited and shat himself at the same time?

This incident was terrifying. How long had this 'family' been doing these things to the point where they saw nothing wrong with it?

This makes me so angry. But I was left in a state of confusion because no one seemed to care. No one apologised. No one wanted the paperwork. No one. Even other neighbours didn't want to get involved because they didn't want trouble at their door. There were dead animals that stunk of bleach. Busted car tyres. Stink bombs. Harassment. Threats. I even woke up one night, hearing something I feel sick to talk about involving her underage daughter. Police weren't interested in another council estate girl besides I had to prove it, how did I know? A housing officer just asked me if she said 'no' at any time during the whole ordeal. They could say they were in love. I was physically paralysed that night. I prayed that what I was hearing wasn't real. I just lay there crying silently hoping not to wake my little sister. I didn't want her to hear it. I faced the police alone to report it. I was so scared and confused that I mustn't have explained it properly because if I had, something would have been done. Right?

I can only tell you my side of the story. Why didn't anyone care? Those kids needed to be saved. I didn't say it properly. I didn't...I wasn't aware of how. No one was surprised. I didn't explain it properly. Stupid bitch, always doing that. Write it down. The police lady called me stupid. The voices would agree.

I'm wrong. People weren't saved because of me. Are you still here?

We lost family during this period. We lost much-loved pets too. Magnified feelings but we were already drained. I don't recall marking any of those moments. Couldn't cry because they'd laugh...

My youngest brother was also in the children's hospital after a burst appendix. They found that funny, while the 'nosy neighbour' told people, even my parents, that it was trivial. "Is that all?" Bitch! We nearly lost a great human being and a nice brother.

I feel more lonely now. While these things went on, I forgot to live. People my age are usually in long-term relationships and have kids of their own...I can't even look at people anymore. I'm back in the corner. Don't look at me. Up close, you will see all my many faults, I can be ugly. But one thing is for damn sure...I do not hurt good people. I love to hurt bad people! There is nothing better than giving bullies a taste of their own medicine! I just don't give a fuck if that offends you, politicians, doctors, housing officers, nosy neighbours or holier than thou 'Hug a Hoodie' trend followers. You want to give bullies, muggers, murderers, criminal thugs, and anti-social nasties a hug? Please live next door to them. Send your vulnerable children, who are still working out who they are, to school with them. Tell your abuser, both young and old, whether their abuse is physical or mental, working and unemployed, and fit or disabled 'I understand'. If you want taxpayer's money, use charity funds to pay for courts, solicitors, criminal damage, and compensation to people who just need to be told affirmatively, and reinforced, that you love them, do it. You live with them, you kind and misinformed wonderful people. God help you because no other fucker will. When did we turn into a society of helping bad people more than good people?

Robin Hood would be pissed. Punishing the real victims, the ones being abused, is now normal? Rewarding the bad with time, attention and understanding, is the measure of how kind people are. It's like walking past *Oliver Twist* lying on the floor in pain, and asking the cruel pickpocket if they need help. Real good people are being ignored, silenced and intimidated into saying nothing because speaking up costs time and money in the short-term, and laws, and community safety (if people speak out), are not the done thing. Not PC.

I won't think too loudly. The voices remind me of everything. They told me they would stay after the bad neighbours left because they didn't want me to have a life. I don't deserve one. But I won't let them make me different from who I am. I offered to take the blame in exchange for them to leave my family out of it.

Please tell everyone I'm sorry. Maybe I can help better in the next life.

The Voices: lifelong assholes. The voices seemed to speak in time to the sounds of the boiler, fans, washing machine, and hoover. They progressed from familiar voices to voices I don't recall. I began hearing my own voice, a voice, in my own head expressing my thoughts and feelings. Nowhere to hide. No privacy. I would hear many people screaming in the background. The voices would tell me what others were doing when I wasn't there. They used vocabulary I didn't know. They even pretended to be kids, even though their vocabulary was well past its use by date, claiming I was a 'monster', a paedophile. I was terrified and vomiting.

I challenged them. Called them out. They were as yellow as a popular rubber duck! Still are. They said they were real. Then stand in front of me and say those things! They, claiming to be police officers, not only outnumbered me but also didn't have the guts to say those horrific things to my face. Me? Quiet, polite, hardworking me? Really?

This was going on while I carried on working and the bad neighbours would harass me with the excuse that their solicitor was nearby. I could have been fired for reacting to them. We also had a massive influx of shoplifters and pickpockets. Which I took personally. Getting the feeling that someone is desperate to hurt me. Bastards. By hurting me, they also hurt everyone around me.

After a couple of months, I'd started mumbling to myself at work as I argued with the voices. Strange looks. But I persevered in being polite, kind and responsive to my colleagues (work family), my customers (mostly regulars), and the temps I trained on the Sundays on the run-up to Christmas.

The voices said they saw me in the shower. Then one night, I was raped, I mean I wasn't physically raped. They told me what they were doing then afterwards told me they were speaking to someone else with my name. How could I tell anyone? I always handled my own problems until then. Probably why I'm so popular. Asking for help made me weak; made the bad people win. I am not a carpet for crappy people who have no guts to admit they have, they are, the problem.

I will take the blame if it is my fault. Hence:

1 wanted bad people to be punished.

I was responsible for pushing my family to keep going when they were on their last straw because it felt like no one was helping. I should have taken time off work. Instead, I made mistakes that meant my 'work family' had to work harder to pick up the pace. I stopped having a life because I'd worry about my family at home. I chose it. My family is worth that.

I can never find the right words to make people understand.

That's why I have been bullied and abused.

I became almost silent – my choice.

I trusted people who showed me kindness.

I hate myself! So fuck off! You want to? Back of the queue voices/bad people!

I am a coward for never standing up to people who claim to be sorry.

I am sorry I bore you!

I am sorry you find me ugly/difficult to stomach.

I haven't told you more personal information out loud.

I chose a barren, loveless existence.

Intake of breath.

What did you choose?

Did you help?

Who are you?

Why the hell are you here?

Clearly, it must be me. I'm wrong. Someone tell me what to do because I feel like I've tried everything, including not complaining. Tried being nice? No. Tried ignoring it? No. Tried standing up to them? No. Tried being angry? No. Tried being honest? No. Tried being like them? Not a chance in hell. I've even tried being a 'pain in the arse' or me duale de culo, freakin' loved it!

So that's what I chose a long time ago. Being me…wait…I chose that? I CHOSE THAT! So I annoy the shit out of all the voices. Little victories keep me going.

Over the years, my internal neighbours have surprised me. They do listen to my thoughts, and my memories, and put up with my really weird personality. They know me more than anyone under my 'family umbrella'. So despite some really nasty and painful conversations they do, on occasion, they surprise me with insightful comments and conclusions. They keep me company so I'm never alone. I love it. They are now brutally honest with me. I like that. I prefer it to pity. They teach me things, I hope I reciprocate. Human behaviour is only one facet, which we can see, hear, and predict. Mental behaviour is another.

Mental behaviour consists of following a habit of thoughts and emotions that then, in turn, influence our actions and habits. We cannot see these or hear them…That's where my voices come in.

Looking for correlations (similarities) between our actions and our life events (experiences) can't accurately be signs of mental illness. It's like saying that if you don't get on with your mum, you will be more likely, more prone to depression.

Is that true? Why? If a psychiatrist claims this in their books, does that make it accurate? Is it simply because this particular event (arguing with your mum) is something a majority of depressives have in common? Is it a subconscious need of the psychiatrist to blame their depression on other people?

Mental behaviour is about why you hold on to specific events (arguing with Mum), why you are reminded of the event (what externally makes you remember, like seeing a mum and son fight in public), and what emotions you feel remembering and witnessing now. What is the result? What physical action is produced? Can others see your responses or do you appear emotionless and motionless?

Simple as that, I think.

The voices have worked on me for many years now. They measure my responses to positive and negative stimuli. I know. They are aggressive and unyielding in their pursuit to 'break' me over and over again. I worry it might kill me. However, I think I understand them sometimes too.

My life was ruined by those neighbours and myself.

My family didn't want to "move the problem on". We didn't want anyone else to suffer. We did it for as long as we could. I was done. Just fucking kill me. Those people took my youth, my confidence, my home, and my feeling of safety.

Schizophrenia – the voices are the only ones that hear me anymore.

Some things should be left in the dark.

For Future Reference to Others That Have Bad Neighbours Affecting Their Mental Health:

Trust with information that everyone on the outside of the problem can communicate and advise with each other. The housing, schools, child services, police and the NHS, all need to share, at their discretion, information crucial to a faster outcome. Why?

Don't assume. Someone is lying for different reasons. Double-check everything they say and record the reasons for believing it is true or false. It also helps if the case goes to court. The more details, the less they need to ask. Just because they have medical appointment letters doesn't mean that they attended it or had anything wrong with them.

Improve community relations. Support is vital to tackle problems on estates. Stop being seen as the enemy. Have the community trust you more than the criminals. This gives bad people nowhere to hide. Involve the community, if they know there's a problem, make them feel indispensable. If people help, knowing they will be rewarded with safety, and given responsibility, they will fight harder for peace of mind. It makes them feel important/crucial.

Offer help to communities by providing a continued presence as a show of solidarity. Making criminals move continuously slows the rise in crime. They need familiar, safe territory where they know escape roots. If you know more than they do, you are a step ahead. Meaning you can funnel them right into your arms. Keeping the pressure on them means their mask will slip, they cannot watch every exit; with larger numbers (people in the communities), you will have more eyes to watch more exits.

Don't pretend you're in control, be in control.

Information gives control. Criminals know all they need to know and they laugh because you "have to feel for them". They know you have to respect their human rights, who protects the human rights of the victim? Is no one allowed to show favouritism to a victim? Don't be confused! Know your job. Check every detail of their story, and know their routine. Missing something? Find it. Earn respect.

Addiction, mental illness, and socio-economic backgrounds are not reasons, they are by-products. Even on drugs, you know stealing/mugging is wrong. Illness has nothing to do with it. Is it wrong? Yes. Don't do it!

"They're only kids!" What about the kids they've hurt, abused, killed? The pensioner that doesn't leave a home where they no longer feel safe? A shop worker whose job is at risk because of shoplifting/threats of abuse? If you feel so bad for the problem kids, then 'save them'. Get them to another place where they won't harm others or themselves. They can learn to be respectful, productive, and happier people. They won't learn if they are not told they were wrong. They won't feel remorse for never being in the shoes of the victim. They get more love, attention, and money for being a problem. In the meantime, how many of you reading this thought about what helps the victims of these wayward kids?

In short, stop passing the problem!

Is it a police matter? A housing matter? Social services? A dispute between neighbours? Domestic Abuse? Who is responsible?

We are all responsible including the perpetrator. Many hands make light work. Working against each other only helps the abuser. Talk and think long-term.

Unfortunately, violence is commonplace these days. Mental abuse is a trend. Emotional bacchanal is expected. We are all at risk of mental illness.

Someone once told me that fear was the only deterrent against abusers. The fear of god. To make someone so scared of the punishment that they are deterred from committing a heinous act of any kind.

Why have we forgotten this principle?

God, in his many forms and names, appears in desperate times to protect the good and terrify the bad. No one fears the wrath of God anymore? So no one fears punishment?

I hear cries of 'to fix bad people we need to understand them, help them, to prevent them from committing the same crimes'. How noble. How kind. How forgiving. How naive. How patronising for their victims.

Politicians, our local members of parliament, condone the mistreatment of those less fortunate and base their knowledge on party supporters' views or books and statistics. Reliable sources, a trusted narrative?

Please, visit all of your constituents. Even those who don't vote. Time and money? Restrictions? Surely if you believe the narratives you are spinning, you will spend time (albeit without overtime) to find solutions to social problems that will come to the forefront in communities with problems big as well as small. Don't believe what others tell you. Go into all of these communities, even dangerous ones, with the protection that ordinary people don't have, and find solutions, not theories.

If it were up to me, I'd have them living in said communities for a month…Did you just panic? If it is so easy to solve, then why did you panic? If you know that noble intentions and kindness would make people safer, have at it. Fix them. You are obviously more qualified; you've read things, met people, and discussed them.

There are good people struggling and you are being put in a position of trust. Listen to everyone. Help those who have the power to help others and stop laughing at victims. That is a politician. That is a leader.

Mental illness is a massive problem. Anxiety and depression are the result of work environments, living environments, and social interactions. Maybe if our MPs didn't have a pay rise every year but generously donated that amount to NHS, police, and pensioners (take your pick), the people would respect you.

Should schizophrenics be allowed to vote? Yes. We are still a minority and British citizens. Every vote counts because we are part of the makeup of Britain. To not vote would be like choosing only white Christians to vote. Are any of us of 'sound mind'? "We can't let the Liverpudlians vote because they are all criminals and crazy people. Oh, and the 'poor' aren't educated enough to make the right decision."

I harbour no prejudice towards anyone except 'bad people'. The 'people' whose words and actions infringe on public safety.

Did you just scoff at that?

Why Are You Doing This Schizo?

Speak up or continue to be a victim.

It's 'none of your business' what your neighbours do.

Whose 'business' is it?

It isn't your responsibility.

Yet no one else will 'step up'. Will anyone help me?

It's none of their business either. Why do it?

Why do I keep fighting?

So you admit it, you instigated the problem. You made yourself, your family, and your other neighbours part of the problem.

Whose problem?

Everyone else's problem. They were dragged into a problem. You made escape unavoidable. Kept them committed.

So you admit, there is a problem?

Okay. Why won't people go to court?

Everyone has reasons.

Reasons or excuses?

So, they should be involved.

You could be putting them in the firing line. You could be making their lives more difficult. Even escalating the problem and creating others. Those people have more important things to think about, why don't you have other things in life to occupy you?

I didn't want to cause other people problems. I know the police, the housing, the MP and their staff have other causes, but they hurt me and my family. They hurt other people's kids. They lied to various people for monetary gain and avoided prosecutions by being anti-social.

Is that all? Anti-social? That's happening everywhere. All of those people have bigger problems and more physical crime issues in poorer areas. The people on those estates need help. They risk their own safety to report crimes. You're more entitled than them?

I don't want to make them more problems, I want them to be part of the solution. If my problem is so trivial, it should be a quick fix. Why focus all of your resources in one place? How can you solve 'bad estates' if you cannot prevent or protect the territory you have? How do we maintain the peace? Or do we take all our resources and move to the next problem area? Isn't that moving the problem around?

Poor area, high crime = low stock value, cheap land. By moving problem people/families to more moderate areas, housing becomes cheaper as crime is then more reported. So we can now say, "This bad area has seen a major drop in crime. Well done, police, well done, housing." Not their fault they rely on rewards, pay-outs, and jobs. But if we solve the problem, jobs are cut in both sectors and the only people who gain anything are the property owners and superior officers. They get accolades. Everyone else gets so many years knocked off their lives. We need to listen to the whispers over the shouts. Sorry. I mean help us to make our neighbourhoods feel safe for us, for you, the elderly, and the kids. It may not seem important but it is. Even criminals don't want to live with criminals because they know how bad it can be.

What about the 'bad people/families' and their mental Illnesses, their ongoing problems?

They should still take responsibility for their actions. I'm schizo. That label shouldn't mean that my concerns for the safety of others should make me a 'liar', dangerous or unable to tell right from wrong.

So mental illness isn't a 'get out of jail free card'. We still know the difference. As labels are prejudicial anyway, take that out of the equation. Just look at the problem for what it is. If a bad thing has happened, then answer accordingly. The problem, who did it, why it was done, did they know it was wrong, evidence to support that (not future evidence, present evidence), and brainstorming of solutions between those investigating. We need long-term solutions. How much money does it cost for housing companies to pursue anti-social tenants? How much does it cost the emergency services and NHS to treat and investigate victims and perpetrators of crimes? How much in medicines and mental health treatments for victims, police officers, perpetrators and bystanders young and old? We cannot net zero those figures but in the long term, we can limit them. For a better society, that's a bargain. Everyone loves a bargain.

What about false reporting of crimes?

As a schizophrenic?

That's one example.

Apologies, genuine remorse should be noted and punishment, if they find no crime was committed, should be made public.

But, you're vulnerable. You have a mental illness.

It's not the voices in my head that made the choice. People can appear sincere and goad you into a reaction. But I chose that action.

Do you think you're better than others? You're very 'preachy'.

I'm better than the 'bad people' you are trying to protect.

You have had more opportunities in life. Those 'bad people/families' have had it hard financially, abusive upbringings, addictions, lack of education etc.

Who told you that? Them?

They have endured a 'hard life'. Can't you, your community understand this? They need help, not punishment.

Maybe I haven't told you everything bad I've experienced in my life. Don't assume because I made some good choices, that I have lived a life of fewer problems than them. They don't need help to choose right from wrong. Are they telling the truth about the abuses they went through? Why let their kids go through the same thing? Why make everyone around them suffer with them?

Most criminals have mental issues.

Most criminals are men.

You're being a pious bitch again.

That is an assumption. There are schizo killers out there. There are even more with no history of schizophrenia. There is even stuff on YouTube about business executives who are successful because they are Sociopaths. What makes criminals notorious and beyond redemption is 'no remorse'. How many people say sorry and mean it to their victims/ survivors?

How many angry people care?

We need emotional and mental stability. If you think a person has mental health issues, reach out, and find them help. Be brave and ask. They don't throw you in a 'loony bin' as soon as you tell them that you hear things, have suicidal thoughts, addictions. Please keep trying. It's when you stop trying that the world becomes more intimidating.

You're appealing to their better nature? Well, professionals have an obligation to care for everyone. We will listen. You are not alone.

I am!

Shut it, Caroline!

(Shouts of annoyed agreement)

Shut up voices! Well…we all get a little shut up inside sometimes.

Shut up…

Unable to escape…

Shut up, CAROLINE!

Squashed together in a tight bowling ball. Struggling to breathe in…

SHUT UP!

We need to…

RIGHT! That is it! CAROLINE!? What?

SHUT UP! (En masse)

Okay! I just want to explain that mental health, Income, disability, race, gender, religion, and language are not factors that influence or impair our morals. They are used as excuses and symptoms/results of other problems. We all know right and wrong. There is no confusion. If someone did that to you, what would you do? Do you want to live in a safe community? How do 'we' do that?

Long-term versus short-term? We can understand that. So how do we 'help' those 'bad people/families' conform?

Punish 'bad' actions and reward 'good people' who call them out truthfully. Move the 'bad people/families' in with other 'bad people'. A taste of their own medicine. For the people who help deal with the 'bad people', inform them, rally communities, or go to court; these 'good' people should be rewarded. Move them to a safer community, and get them financial help for all the days, times, and sacrifices that they've made to make communities safer. Reward 'good' employees, officers etc., for the extra care and trust and time they sacrifice to aid all communities.

And that will help 'bad people' to 'conform'?

Yes. People love rewards. They have to see as well as read or hear about the benefits of being good.

You are a depressing schizo. Why should anyone believe what a mentally ill person has to say? Why should the police believe a schizo is reporting a real crime? It's all in your head. No one else saw or heard it. You're hallucinating.

So a 'criminal' is innocent until proven guilty?

So a 'victim' is a liar until proven innocent?

Reporting a crime that didn't happen would ruin lives and reputations...

Including the victims?

Providing we identify the real victims.

But you won't know unless you look. If it is true, there will be evidence somewhere. Don't give up! Don't stop trying when people need you! Don't reduce whether a person/family can feel safe, down to money!

You're being melodramatic again...

I find it difficult to find the right words. I used to read a lot. A lot. I can't stop explaining. People don't understand or feel the same...I need to describe it. Please understand.

The Pros of Our Modern World

We are fortunate enough to live in an age where more information is accessible to more people or someone's pet cat called bonkers that shadow boxes.

Our schools are better equipped with tech unless you live in a good community where teachers huddle in a dark corner playing on a Gameboy. Hey, Tetra was an awesome spy tool and addictive.

We are in a world where our leaders and representatives can and are ready to speak up about the things we'd usually try to ignore, praying that it will never happen close to home...

If you are prepared to talk about a problem in society to others, then you must have ideas/solutions to share too, right? Otherwise, you're just complaining.

Swap political correctness for 'normal life'.

Investing in a country's future long-term instead of short-term easy solutions. It's just putting multiple plasters on a broken bone. It'll hold for now. Let another doctor fix it down the line.

Make no mistake, the world is changing constantly, making decisions should be given to those who care.

The transition from illness to health depends upon not just a doctor's knowledge but also on the experience (details/symptoms) of the patient and the input of those who are around them every day.

To my fellow mentally ill out there: Let the storm in your minds rage on and trust those with wings to shelter you,

I am a schizo that probably bothers the police more than others. I understand if they don't like me. I understand that I may anger them. I am sorry. I just wanted to help the 'Good guys'. Better safe than sorry.

An Overview of My Life and the World I Grew In

I was born in Fazakerley Hospital, Liverpool, Merseyside at the beginning of the 1980s. It was a dark-looking future.

Unemployment, closing businesses, and the beginnings of a drug epidemic on estates would shape the fortunes of every generation that followed. The economic north/south divide was obvious to many. We felt alone. A scouser alone? Never.

Despite our woes, we survived on laughter and shared experiences. I'm sure that if you search the internet, you will find details of criminal gangs and the Toxteth riots. Did any of these things factor into my subsequent schizophrenia and depressive state now? I don't think so...but I think that it explains my coping mechanisms.

If you don't laugh, you cry! So laugh with people, not at people.

Growing up, I don't remember anyone discussing any mental health things. Never heard the words autism, depression, or schizophrenia. Never. But I was a kid, a little kid. So I asked my mum. She said, "It wasn't a subject for conversation". In fact, she doesn't remember anyone talking about this stuff when she was a kid either.

Other kids and adults who behaved differently or had difficulties concentrating or communicating were called 'stupid' and 'backward' by kids and their parents. Nobody explained these people. People either ignored them or 'took the piss'. My family either ignored my breakdown or felt I was responsible for driving them to theirs. They were angry and said they didn't recognise me as me anymore. I felt ostracised. Am I me?

Police distrust grew and they were seen as the enforcers of a Thatcher government that didn't care. Thatcher left kids hungry, and parents angry. Instead of thieving what we needed, taking handouts from churches, taking jobs from drug dealers that the government couldn't provide, knowing your kids couldn't get good jobs because families couldn't send the kids to college or university, and never being told of any choices we had caused a shit load of mental health problems and addictions. Alcohol and substance abuse were escapist coping mechanisms for many.

Nearly all my friends from infants and juniors were from homes with addiction and abuse. Single-parent families were rampant in certain estates. People who were honest about everything in their lives (including addictions) were 'made an example of'. Those who lied and blamed others who had similar situations were thrown money and sympathy. Short-term solutions for long-term abusers who get rewarded instead of reaping what they sow.

I have little idea of the world around me. Looking back, I had multiple breakdowns over things I found difficult in life. Yet over the years, my thoughts were always thinking. Questions, answers, more questions. Explaining, always explaining. Finding reasons for everything that posed questions. I want to understand. Because whatever is wrong then I can fix it. If I can fix it, I can ask the question and share the solution. Good foundations, strong foundations mean I won't keep breaking and you won't break. Still looking.

TEEN YEARS

"Can I beat you up?"

I was asked that question.

"Want those lads over there to fancy us." It's not funny.

They are asking my permission to beat me up. So they don't feel responsible. They don't care. They don't care? Smell that?

King Kong's first dump of the day!

What? Too common and crude? I find farts hilarious too. If I have offended you, I am sorry. Truly. My only intention was to make you smile or laugh. This stuff is tough to read. It felt tougher to live it. A moment of being happy…to escape, keeps what is left of me together.

"Liar."

"Sad bitch."

"Morticia Adams."

"Milk bottle."

"Why are you so pale? What's wrong with you?"

"Who'd go out with you?"

Not just my fellow high schoolers getting to know me. Unsurprisingly, some teachers and family said one or two of those things too.

Lads that enjoyed humming the 'Sweeney Family' theme tune, a variant of the Adams Family theme tune. For some, it was a hobby for after school and at weekends when Mum, my brothers and my little baby sister would walk to Nan's house for a visit. Standing in a group smirking, pulling faces at my sister in her pushchair, and swearing in our faces. WHY?

I am the common denominator. Something must be wrong with me. WHAT? The majority of teachers throughout my life described me as courteous, very quiet, and bright. A few employed the same phrase, "A pleasure to teach". I never ever hurt anyone with intention. I hate bullies and teachers who claim that I should 'feel sorry for them' and that these abusers are 'the real victims'. I'm the problem?

I need to change my attitude. I should be more understanding "Bullying doesn't happen in this school" "You're just oversensitive".

Just "kids being kids".

Kids, all kids, are developing their personalities, and their beliefs, especially in their teens. Who are they? Who will they be?

What's their outlook on the world and others in it going to be?

If your child strips another of their confidence for any stupid reason, including 'just not liking them', who is responsible for that?

Your children understand the world through your teachings and your beliefs. They watch you to see how to react to the people around them. Do you accept responsibility? Do you want your child to be a bully? What morals have you taught? If you have made bad decisions as a parent, admit it! Tell your child you did wrong. Tell your child's victim what your child did was wrong. Tell their worried family you were wrong. Apologise. Then promise your child you will be better for them because you love them and want them to be happy but taking our frustrations out on others that have not hurt them is wrong. Work with teachers to get both pupils' help.

Treat others how you want to be treated.

Stop punishing victims. Stop throwing money at bad people. Reward victims. Be honest with them. Reward those who prove they feel genuine remorse.

Talking in my head to my voices. We challenge perceptions. My voices know almost everything about me. Makes me feel naked. I have nowhere to hide, to escape, to avoid. While they may not provide closure to problems in my life, they provide an arena to face my fears and help me see my fears from another perspective.

How can our members of parliament help?

Legislation: The Mental Health Act of 1983 gave us much-needed rights to refuse hospital permission.

We need to have complaints of abuse by prejudiced members of the community, a hate crime.

People of any disability who are ridiculed, abused, and targeted in any community should be considered 'vulnerable'. Do not dismiss negative behaviour by others as acceptable, as "just kids being kids" or "it is your word against theirs". Everyone matters even if some cannot understand that. Observe cautionary discretion.

Protection and connection.

Free internet by prescription: A once-a-year payment policy/licence for the vulnerable. That is the elderly and the vulnerable. Including those who are affected by certain crimes. Providing an essential lifeline for adults and children who need to talk to people to know they aren't alone in the world. Could it work through charities?

Be human: Members of parliament should include more local charities and mental health services like the Early Intervention Team and show they want to help everyone. Everyone should be Included.

School policies: Train teachers to recognise and support colleagues and students at risk. Make certain that it is the responsibility of parents and teachers to record every incident of bullying. The perpetrator and the victim, all should be taken seriously. And provide legislation that protects victims and does not reward (feel sorry for) the victim's abusers.

Parents need to be responsible for their children. Teachers need to be responsible for a child's care during school hours.

Remember: Report every incident. Assure staff that they will not be penalised for the number of reports they have. In fact, keeping records will prove to parents, students and the sly community that this school cares and their children are cared for during school hours.

All abuse is wrong, including hiding it.

More grants for students: For studying mental health and working as volunteers in hospitals, schools, and charities during studies in the final year.

Disability hate crimes: I was unfortunate enough to have a neighbour to whom I had told about my schizophrenia and depression. They told others. I was subjected to months of abuse and when I confronted them, they told me, "It's all in your head", and denied saying anything. I believed the things they said about me. There's something wrong with me, I must be a bad person. Yet for 2–3 years, before they moved into the flat beneath mine, I was happier. I got on well with all my neighbours.

One night at breaking point, I ran from my flat in my pyjamas, nothing else. I ran past my sister, who was asleep in the living room, out the door, and ran to my parents' home. Because of what they were saying about me and to me. They were laughing at me. My sister was upset when she was woken by a door slam.

They denied everything but both my sister and my younger brother heard them. Yet because of my incredibly sensitive state, I didn't tell the police fearing that because I am schizophrenic, I wouldn't be believed.

I was lucky I ran to my parents' home. I was on autopilot. I could just as easily have ended up in the nearby canal.

False or confusing representations in the media of schizophrenics as serial killers or people in strait jackets is degrading. A social 'norm', a fuck up (sorry, just emotional, no offence meant).

I am a quiet individual. I worked, just after I dropped out of university, the same job for over a decade. Always customer friendly, I would also help out at other stores doing the manager's job. I don't bother anyone. I am a published poet and a loving family member (though I have no children of my own). I don't understand people who don't understand. I want my MP to represent all their constituents. I want to know that I still matter. We all matter.

Anything to Pass On?

Yes. I want to haunt the conscience of bullies, teachers, abusers, and enablers, I want them to be afraid. I want their victims to become survivors.

MPs who include and protect all communities deserve loyalty in return for their hard work. MPs like Bill Esterson and their invaluable staff like Veronica Bennett, who never back down from problems either big or small. Their voters are unwavering because no one is forgotten.

To ill-informed social workers and housing officers, could you please do your job thoroughly? It will help you and your colleagues in the long run, create more trust in communities where good people need to be lifted out of bad communities. Question every detail, be prepared, and remember not to be hoodwinked by bad people who feel no remorse.

Can medical professionals please stop procrastinating about mental illnesses? Some think that if you do exactly as they say then you will be cured. And if you aren't, then you are lazy, a scrounger or a really good actor. Well, any professional would truly realise the human mind is complex. We cannot just snap out of it. Unfortunate lifetime prisoners of their own minds and 'professionals' minds do not understand each other...Maybe you need to work that out before we listen.

Could police officers talk to housing associations as well as other charities, and schools, or even start up local YouTube videos? Don't pass the buck by claiming that it's not your problem to already distressed people. Public relations with the police should mean showing locals that the police care, they're reliable, and they are people of their word. If you can't help, at least help by not forgetting them; even if it's by e-mails and visits. If there is red tape, quotas (statistics), or anything that prevents you from doing your job then inform people. We will rally for you to help create laws and policies that benefit the good people who need you.

It will be hectic and time-consuming in the 'short-term' but because of your foresight, the 'long-term' benefits will improve communications and turn the tide of the causes of mental health illnesses. To cure or cope, we all need to be surrounded by positivity, trust and safety.

Right...the voices. Every emotion, thought, and memory I have, that I feel forced to relive – I hate you! However, you all made me mentally confront my worst fears, the worst of myself and gave me nowhere to hide. You(s) know more about me than anyone I have ever met in my entire life. I thought I was a ghost. How did you see me?

A1 – A Problem?

Briefly touching on this subject. Okay, artificial intelligence is the promise of an easier future. Machines doing all the repetitive jobs and eventually cancelling out 'human error'. Making businesses and organisations more cost-effective and efficient...Aha...So what you're saying is that A1 will replace a human worker with or without disabilities?

It will be more efficient, saving companies millions.

In wages?

We don't have to have boring jobs anymore.

So factory and warehouse workers are liberated from employment? Wow! (Sarcasm)

No more annoying phone jobs with difficult customers. No being unable to understand accents.

So call centres here and abroad will become obsolete?

Your profits will go through the roof!

So business owners/shareholders will get even richer?

Just think, no more overheads.

So no pensions, injury insurance, wages, holiday pay, maternity leave pay...

No stealing. No bullying...

No personal touches. No praise...

Think of the money!

Which no fucker, apart from the owners, is going to get!

Don't be a negative nelly.

Don't be a dickhead! So what we get to look forward to is watching the rich spend more money. While ex-workers struggle to find another low-paid job to pay for essentials that the robots will make when they are fired?

Don't hate people who are financially well off. Just because they bettered themselves.

They got to where they are all by themselves. So the workers that worked extra hours without extra pay, the ones that deal with the public on a day-to-day basis even when verbally or physically abused, aren't the reason why people get rich and stay rich? You wouldn't need doctors. AI will solve staffing problems and reach conclusions much quicker. So instead of speaking to a 'human psychiatrist' about my depression or schizophrenia, I will in fact be heard by a synthetic replica of a human mind...I don't know why but that seems ironic.

You wouldn't have to work as a police officer, a factory worker, or a volunteer anymore. Putting yourself in needless danger? Doing a soul-destroying, boring job, for years? Why take mundane or embarrassing jobs to help children, the elderly, or the disabled? Because I want to live! I want to be proud, I want to know that my fellow human beings care, and I want to hone my detective skills and understand 'human behaviour'.

But human error...

Is as inevitable as a robot's. We all break down. Where are the jobs? The wages? How can poor people live? How can benefits and the NHS survive when unemployment and a growing population become overwhelming?

I am preaching, I hope, to the converted. Business owners and investors please think before you buy into the AI dream. What you lose is greater than what you gain. As your bank balance goes up, beware of abandoned employees on the way down.

I Promise I Am Calm Now: Coping Mechanisms?

Coping for yourself or with family:

Maybe stran—

No! No!

Or pro—

No! For God's sake be normal. BE NORMAL!

Write it down: Keep a diary of what you hear or see. Record the day/time and what was heard. Is there a pattern? When are the voices more intrusive? Has it improved or worsened since you started on meds, changed routine etc.?

You do not have to show this to anyone. Sometimes it's just therapeutic to write it down. I would write it down then take a breath and rip it up.

Do what you love: I write, watch TV, or play games if I can concentrate. I am a tech idiot so others usually help me. Go for walks, exercise, and talk. Just find an outlet for yourself. You are still alive, I promise you.

Learn words to your favourite songs: Maybe you have always wanted to learn a difficult song like *'Um Bongo', 'I'm my own grandpa'*, or anything by the Rock and Heavy Metal commune. I want to learn, *'House of the Rising Sun'* and relearn, *'I'm the Scatman'*…don't judge.

This will provide distractions, even if only a short breathing space. Improve cognitive thinking. It will also impress or annoy family and friends…I love it.

Laughter: The best medicine. I like to imagine comic sketches in my head like a hippy with anger issues, a drug-addicted alien with severe withdrawal symptoms, or me in various situations under the duress of Murphy's Law.

Laughing is healthy. Burns calories. Laugh harder, laugh stronger, laugh longer. If people see you laughing alone, then either concentrate on a phone or sod them. Laughing is a good thing, so say hello and give them your kindest smile. Feels nice, doesn't it?

Research schizophrenia: For sufferers and carers. Knowledge is power. Ignorance gives birth to fear. Finding more information lets us know we are not alone. There are others out there.

Hopefully, it will prepare you for long-term success. No surprises.

Listen to your voices: Yep. I said it. It may seem crazy because it is. I am doing that. Why? Because I need the voices to have a reason as to why they talk, I listen, hoping to solve it all. Are they trying to tell us something that needs to be addressed? When you feel ready, ask them.

My voices represent negative memories that I have no closure on. My worst fears manifested. They make avoidance impossible.

These mechanisms are not carved in stone. Find what works for you even if others think otherwise. There is never a single question and never a wrong answer…just those that tried and those that didn't.

How can the wider society help?

End ignorance: Employers need to be given advice to put in place measures to prevent discrimination. Take a staff training day and learn about recognising colleagues with mental illnesses to dispel any bullying. There are charities and organisations that would happily and freely give talks, provide digestible information, and give ideas to help everyone.

Stop whispering: People do hear you whether directly or through word of mouth. It creates an unpleasant work environment. It cannot just isolate workers, it can affect your customer base too and in turn, your workers' morale.

Create new policies: Anti-bullying policies are crucial to the safety of your employees. Show you care. A happier environment is a productive one. Maybe even give a recorded talk yourself on mental health issues. The human touch.

Remember: Your employees/colleagues represent you, and your brand. Reputations are made and broken because of you and your workers. You want people to see you positively and not negatively.

End stigma culture: To not hire someone qualified for the job just because of any health reasons is illegal. However, when you hire or turn down people for positions based on a disability, you don't have to say it is because of their disability…sad fact. You need to ask an honest question and that is, "Can they do the job?" Surely, experience and the benefits a person can bring to the table are the most important things for the future of your company.

How can NHS/police/social services help?

Consistency: I find it difficult to tell people what I see and hear as a schizophrenic. I feel like I am constantly explaining myself to different faces. We need to see regular people, not strangers after strangers. This will build rapport and trust.

From my experience, the mental healthcare system is overloaded. So not just the public are suffering but people who work in emergency services also struggle with mental health problems. Many won't seek help or admit they need it! The staff is overwhclmed. If I struggle to get appointments or struggle to get on waiting lists, A&E will be the nexl stcp but I cannot wait 3–6 hours in a crowded waiting room to talk to someone about suicidal thoughts. We need more funding for much-needed services and the staff that work on them. Charities need to be more involved to alleviate services staff.

Respectful: People with mental health issues are not stupid. We may be less capable of communicating with other people or trusting people with our problems, but we are still human. We have feelings, it's just we can't always express them like other people.

There is a culture of passive bullying in our emergency services. Making fun of your patients or of people reporting a crime because they are genuinely scared should not be allowed to become the 'norm'.

Do not be fooled: Can your officers, your staff, spot a faker? Some people lie to get arrested under the Mental Health Act. Shocking as it may seem! To escape punishment. All crimes and acts of violence should be investigated and that includes access to medical documents for police to establish if they are being lied to. And punish them appropriately.

Attitude: Please do not tell a mental health sufferer of any kind that you know what they are going through. It is patronising and hurtful. Reading a book isn't the same as experiencing it. If you could empathise, that would be amazing and lead to more trust. Sympathy is also welcome for sufferers and carers alike. Lack of patience, not time, should be the enemy. It's okay to not know the ins and outs. Just don't be a jerk!

Please remember: We are really grateful for all your hard work! Even if we forget to say it sometimes. Don't let a few small-minded people ruin things for the rest of you. We all have emotions. Thank you all for your resilience, your kindness, and, most importantly to me, your humour. It is always better to laugh than cry! Thank you!

Please note this is my experience. By the time people read this, things may have changed.

Please do not tolerate 'workplace bullies'. Over the years I have seen tired, overworked police officers, nurses etc., behave miserably and angrily to each other as well as the people, they help. Nobody wants to go to work if their environment is 'toxic'.

Police, for example, get plenty of 'grief' from criminals. Their superiors are also their mentors, role models etc. Define what separates a police officer from a criminal. Be everything you are supposed to represent.

A healthy 'family' atmosphere, rewarding 'good' officers, punishing 'bad' officers, and helping each other are vital for winning the 'popularity war' between police and criminals in local communities. Who are the police? Is there a 'good' officer going unnoticed? The respect from other officers, while not a promotion, is creating encouragement. No 'good' officer should go unnoticed. A great leader brings out the best in people, not put them down.

Stand up for those who can't and raise their confidence levels, self-worth levels, sense of identity and productivity.

You don't try to solve crimes or help people if you're degraded in front of other officers.

How do we tap into a society where there are negative ideas?

Cons of modern society as seen through the eyes of a schizophrenic: Feel free to debate among yourselves and your inner voices.

Unfortunately, bias and prejudices are still commonplace in ALL cultures, and news/media rhetoric is awash with damning criticism of MPs, police, NHS healthcare, and immigration.

Political correctness is a trend for those with nothing to complain about (but it gets you more views).

Racism is directed at every religion, culture, and colour (including white and mixed race).

Environmental piracy is an epidemic amongst corporations that seem to have a monopoly in politics the world over. Influencers connect to people more than 'average' working heroes, like police officers and firemen.

Perfection does not exist! No matter how hard a generation tries to better the world they live in (please don't stop trying).

Distrust will always be in every individual.

We cannot change but we can adapt…to cope.

Am I Who I Think I Am?

I am not a doctor.

I don't work in healthcare.

I am not an influencer.

I don't want fame.

I don't know any police officers.

I know very little about politics.

I'll never be a teacher, or become rich.

Am I who they think I am?

I need to worry less.

I want to give back.

I want a safe home.

I want to know more good people.

I want my own voice.

I need to remain a student or become old.

Who are you?

Hi, I'm Caroline…

Relating
To My Voices?

WTF?

At one point I had so many voices, some claiming to be people I knew, that I couldn't give you a number. It was a 'Hate Caroline Comic Con'. Crowded with males and females.

1. They wanted to recruit me as a child abuser because they were.
2. They told me they were going to, then claimed they raped my little sisters.
3. They said they watched me in the shower.
4. They bombarded me with crowds of screaming people, heartbeats, and threats.
5. They claimed to be the police that were helping the bad neighbours because they were like them. The neighbours would give them sexual pleasure and watch me and my sisters and brothers through a thermal camera.

6. Laughed when I begged them to stop, when they knew I couldn't physically protect the kids, when I poured my heart out and cried myself to sleep.
7. Said they were with the new neighbour.
8. Said they'd leave when I was 45 years old.
9. Claimed they would leave and come back in "three years' time". They never left.
10. Told me I'd always be alone physically.
11. Told me to "go asleep and never wake up".
12. They said they were punching me. I swear I felt it.
13. I promise that I'd seen someone with my name and listed all my characteristics, including my quirks (like WED-NES-DAY, say it as you see it) when I Googled my final name. I even pleaded with my care coordinator to Google my name to show him, to prove it. It was gone. He let me try a few minutes longer to find it, but I failed. I have issues but my personality is the thing that matters to me the most. That is mine. That is me. Why would you take that away from me? Is your own that bad? I spent years trying to come to terms with and love who I am even if other people didn't. I forged my own original path by staying true to myself. These voices, these people tried to kill me and rob me of the fight I had left in me; bury me and take the only thing I'd begun to love.
14. They took my confidence away. Made me self-conscious again. I left my job and now get nervous every time a phone rings or I hear a knock at the door. Back in the corner. Don't look at me because I disgust anyone who notices me.

15. Positive? Brace yourself. During a crappy suicide attempt, one voice, just one, saved me. It's hazy but he shouted at me to stop. So I put the lid back on the bleach, and then Dad suddenly knocked on the bathroom door.

16. They find me funny, not boring. I am a self-confessed 'stupid genius'. I deliberately don't understand and misinterpret words, phrases, and challenge prejudicial views with sarcasm. They find my humour understandable even if they don't agree with my views.

17. They are the only people who have ever called me 'beautiful'. They could be lying but they sounded sincere.

18. They are brutally honest in what they think of me, people around me, themselves and question everyone's honesty.

19. They judge who I am by my own thoughts and actions. They don't judge me based on what others say about me.

20. They talk like psychology students. They understand predictive behaviour even though we are at odds about Freud and the 'self-fulfilling prophecy'. I don't like it either. I don't believe we become what others tell us we are. I believe we become a personality based on experience and the decisions, and choices we make. We all know right from wrong.

21. They are probably more open-minded than me. More accepting of a variety of people, even bad ones.

22. They don't tell me personal details about their lives because I'd probably use it against them in an angry moment.

23. They are the only friends I have. How many people just laughed at that? One too many?

24. Despite myself, I do respect them. Honest! Because they learn from a lot of people, even from each other. Their bond as friends as well as through work is surprising to the point where I...yeah, maybe a bit envious.

25. They know how to press my buttons. I am a reactor. They make me react. Bastards.

A Schizo's Humour: What I Find Funny!

You may have noticed that I laugh sometimes. Say 'weird' things. Sarcasm, un-PC, filthy humour, the unexpected, and the mocking. This has nothing to do with my mental illness; I am that damned funny. That's me...Hi!

I am the person who randomly waves at passers-by. I am the shop assistant who sold designer teddy bears in Maghull simply by playing with them. I even allowed my fellow workers to join in. I am the sister who embarrassed her older brother not knowing if he would laugh or be angry with me (I wanted him to laugh). I am the girlfriend who told the rudest jokes in public houses (I apologise if anyone was offended by that). I am the friend that scared the shit out of gothic people after watching a horror film. I am the random person who challenges your views on life in an unpolitical way to make you consider people differently.

But no one considered me funny as a teen student. It influenced my self-deprecation as a protective humour. The idea is that I take 'the piss' out of myself before 'bad' people do. In fact, I barely laughed at all in those days, let alone smiled.

Humour is always the best medicine even if others don't 'get it'.

People are cruel. Always looking for someone to blame. They can use humour as a deflection because there is so much wrong with them. They won't take responsibility for mistreating others.

Not their fault if "you're weird" or "ugly".

Anyway, laughter is the best exercise I know and I don't know much about exercise. The gym is another world to me.

"C Star Bubble 44, 34, 44. I have arrived in an alien world with what appears to be perfect homo sapiens. Some actually look happy. Water runs down their strangely arousing forms. Metal contraptions that seem to be making them work. I suspect some kind of kinetic energy is involved to power this huge complex that is hidden from the real world…We've been spotted! I hide my curvaceous fuller figure behind a fatter friend(sigh of relief). The danger has passed…"

My comic idols range from Abbott and Costello, Morcombe and Wise, to Rik Mayall and Adrian Edmondson. Lee Evans is a comic genius. Which I am sure he appreciates from the mentally ill. I even have a crush on all these comedians, as well as admire their confidence and audacity.

I have noticed that people don't believe schizophrenics should have any emotions. Or perhaps, sick crazies with a (sick) sense of humour. What is this based on?

(a) Smarter people: Doctors, nurses, the news.

(b) Influential people: Politicians, Nobel prize winners, YouTubers.

(c) The internet: Wikipedia, Google, Facebook.

(d) Personal Experience: Family members, colleagues, neighbours.

(e) An actual person with mental health problems: Doctors, nurses, police, politicians, teachers, family, friends, neighbours.

Do people talk about who they know? What they've researched? How are these conclusions reached? Are they accurate, truthful, and without error? The answer? There is no finite, written-in-stone, solution. We are learning all the time. Thank God! How open-minded we are! Are we not looking for the unexpected anymore? Are there no mysteries about the human mind?

Don't assume, please. I admire people in all those fields that care, are emotional, challenging, learning, and curious.

Why do we have to be so serious in stressful jobs/situations? Humour helps us cope. Cope with fear, awkwardness, sadness and celebrate happy times with good people. It's not wrong to make life easier, and more productive, letting us all cope even in difficult times. Just don't do it at the expense of others.

Wouldn't cops be more dedicated to the job if they laughed together, not just be depressed together?

Sitting in a van waiting to do a dawn raid on criminal gangs, the tension is so palpable that no one speaks. What if one just farted? What if someone released the tension like that? Like their spirit trumpeting in nervous agreement to the task ahead. And if it smells, shouldn't we acknowledge that?

Shouldn't the team leader crack a smile before he lets in the fresh air? Shouldn't they run focused into the gang's den safe in the knowledge that it couldn't smell worse than what they just experienced? Shouldn't they?

Things like this bring people together against a common enemy.

Respect! Show the good guys some love and Febreze. Seriously, what did you eat?

Police don't want to be laughed at. It's a serious job. (Silence)

But if people are tired and unhappy, are they productive? Will the job be concluded quickly if they work long hours?

Quality versus quantity. And medical professionals? Psychiatrists? They are crucial whether their patients work or not. Why are we seeing a mental health crisis?

Money.

The cause, symptoms, quality, and quantity of life. But we can't save everyone.

Well, hopefully, by saving a life, that life will take your lessons and apply it to others. One person at a time is better than no one at all. At least when you meet your God on judgement day you can honestly say, "I tried to help everyone that crossed my path". And schizos that report a crime? Aren't you wasting their time? Time is money.

I already explained it, didn't I?

Temper.

I don't report a crime for attention. I report a criminal act that I have witnessed to the proper authorities. I am a schizo, not a 'liar'. How will you know if it's the truth if you don't investigate?

Stop stigmatising schizophrenics!

A sense of humour, hey?

Don't label people by their disabilities, where they are from, how much money they have, or where they worship. Don't make it statistic based e.g. 80% of crimes reported by schizophrenics are false. Wasting 'x' amount of time and 'x' amount of money. So we tend to ignore schizos. What if we're right? 20% of crimes are real. Good. Can you afford to ignore a member of the public willing to talk to you about 'x' amount of victims that have no voice?

Too serious. I'm bored…I'm gonna wee myself.

I peed myself once…I was scared. Funny.

Schizophrenic emotion is like being on an old rollercoaster. Highs, lows, fear, adrenaline, and then extreme quiet (you feel but are unable to show it). This ride is not for everyone. The foundation track with twists, turns, and loops is confusing but it has to come to an end. Until then, the lights are bright, the music is annoying, the queues are long, and the sights are new.

Someone take a picture while we are happy.

As all too soon we move on…

Caroline? That's not funny.